PERFECT MASSAGE THERAPY

THE BEST MASSAGE TIPS YOU WISH YOU KNEW

JAMIE J.

CONTENTS

Introduction v

1. The Erogenous Zones 1
2. Sensual Massage in sex therapy 4
3. How is Sensual Massage done? 6
4. Beginners Guide to Sensual Massage 8
5. Gels and Oils used for Sensual Massage 11
6. Sensual Massage Techniques 13
7. Advanced Sensual Massage 16

Sneak Peek - Chapter 1 19

©Copyright 2022 – All rights reserved by Jamie J.

The content of this book may not be reproduced, duplicated, or transmitted without direct written permission from the author or publisher.

ISBN-978-1-63970-130-8

Legal Notice:

This book is copyright protected. This is only for personal use. You cannot amend, distribute, sell, use, quote, or paraphrase any part of the content within this book without the consent of the author or publisher.

Disclaimer notice:

Please note the information contained within this document is for educational and entertainment purposes only.

Every attempt has been made to provide accurate, up-to-date, and reliable complete information.

No warranties of any kind are expressed or implied. Readers acknowledge that the author is not engaging in the rendering of legal, financial, medical or professional advice. The content of this book has been derived from various sources. Please consult a licensed professional before attempting any techniques outlined in this book.

By reading this document, the reader agrees that under no circumstances is the author responsible for any losses, direct or indirect, which are incurred as a result of the use of the information contained within this document, including, but not limited to, -errors, omissions, or inaccuracies.

 Created with Vellum

INTRODUCTION

Sensual Massage is direct stimulation of the outer and inner layers of the muscles and tissues of the body using different techniques. It helps heal the tissues and develops a sense of well-being and relaxation. The term 'massage' is directly borrowed from the French word massage, and an examination of the word's root around the globe (Arabic 'massa', Greek 'masso', Latin 'massa') would reveal that the term means dough or knead and you get to see a lot of kneading movements in Massage.

Massage involves the movement of hands or different parts of the body or a mechanical tool over the body at various degrees of pressure, movements, tension, or vibration on another body. It can benefit the whole body or part of it or various internal organs.

Over the years, Massage has gained the reputation of being a cure for many ailments and also as a lifestyle for many around the globe.

Sensual Massage is a pleasurable variation of this technique in which the body's erogenous zones are massaged. This helps in arousal and even enhances sexual performance and health. This is not anything new as the health benefits of sexual or sensual Massage have been known and practiced for a long time. While the main area of focus in sensual Massage for males is the genital area, it also includes their breasts. Genital Massage may also be termed mutual masturbation.

This is a part of therapy, foreplay, or even post-sex.

Sensual Massage, unlike Traditional Massage, appeals to all senses. This is what makes it unique and what needs to be noted:

1. The eyes
2. The ears
3. The nose
4. The palate
5. The skin

In Traditional Massage, only the skin is tended to. However, as the other sense are also to be taken care of in Sensual Massage, there needs to be a set procedure of preparations.

The ambiance is of prime importance. This will take care of three senses by itself.

The room should be warm to the feel and the sight. A fireplace is the best place to indulge in a Sensual Massage or a warm-colored room with red or orange paint or curtains. The light should primarily come from candles, or the electrical bulbs downed to a dim shimmer.

You can use scented candles and ambergris or incense sticks that are not overpowering and don't smoke the room. Light and soft music played at a soft volume also add to the relaxing of the body and mind. The eyes, nose, and eras are tended to at just the ambiance alone.

Food also plays a very important part in Sensual Massage. It may range from sweet red wine to dry fruits or dates and grapes. Some people also take elaborate courses like spicy roasted meat and bread in small portions. If you use spicy foods, remember to clean your mouth and hands completely with mild soap.

Unlike Traditional Massage, you are not limited to any part of the body, and you can touch the intimate parts. But be sure that your partner enjoys your touch. It is more about giving than receiving, so make it a point to let your partner know that you would like to gift something special. It is also good to leave the room while your partner gets undressed and have a sheet to cover themselves with. Never rush anything, and it's good to not have an aim when indulging in a Sensual Massage.

Sensual Massage is a good way to build trust among partners and deepen the bonds that you already have. It makes you feel better in your intimate moments and understand true relationships. It takes lovemaking to a level that you make 'love' and bring on newer meanings to your intimate relations. Some exercises even let you feel connected so deep that you feel as if your souls are connected. It also lets you feel less ashamed and revel in your nudity in front of your partner.

1

THE EROGENOUS ZONES

The term is taken from the Greek Eros, meaning love, and Genes meaning born. Therefore, the term applies to any part of the body that has a level of sensitivity at a heightened level as there are several nerve endings. The stimulation of these parts directly or indirectly produces sexual arousal, fantasies, and even orgasm.

Erogenous zones are spread all over the body. Some areas are more sensitive than others. Depending on the body, stimulation of these parts can produce different arousal levels. To give a sensual massage, a thorough understanding of the erogenous zones is essential as an immediate orgasm may often reduce the effects of the massage.

The Erogenous zones are divided into two categories:

1. Nonspecific Zones: These areas resemble normal skin and have a lot of nerve endings that help in heightened

stimulation. The nape of the neck, inner arms, etc. are some examples.
2. Specific Zones: These areas are denser in nerve endings and often cause sexual arousal. It is said that they have a close connection with the brain and the brain's reward system.

For males, the focus falls on the pubic region mainly. The erogenous zones are the areas like the top part of the glans and the sides, the side of the penis, the scrotum, the perineum, the anus, and the surrounding areas.

There are many more erogenous zones when it comes to women. The genital area of women is called the vulva. The clitoris and the outer parts of the vagina have a lot of nerve endings and can be stimulated even to reach an orgasm without penetration.

Other erogenous areas include:

1. The Scalp: A massage to the scalp or a hair caress is relaxing and yet very stimulating to many.
2. The nape of the neck is a very sensitive part and is usually aroused by kissing, biting (softly), or licking. It is an extremely sensitive zone in females and where 'love bites' are found.
3. The Ear: The outer sides of the ear and the lobe are sensitive areas that respond to licking or nibbling.
4. The Chest: The entire breast area of both men and women has several nerve endings and can be aroused using the hands. The areola and the nipples are also

highly sensitive. Stimulating the hair around the areola produces oxytocin and stimulates the genital region.
5. The Abdomen: The lower part of the abdomen and the entire navel is very responsive to touch. They also stimulate the genital areas primarily due to their proximity.
6. The Arms: The softer inner parts of the arm and your elbow are extremely erogenous to both men and women.
7. The Armpits: This is a highly erogenous area, especially if it has hair on it. Slowly caressing the armpit is a very stimulating experience, and it is also believed to produce pheromones in men and women.
8. The Fingers: The fingers, especially the tips and the top cone, have an abundance of nerve endings and can be stimulated orally.
9. The Legs: The inner part of the thighs leading to the pubic region is very responsive to caresses and light massages.
10. The Feet: Especially the toes as there are a lot of nerve endings, responds to caresses and oral stimulation. The rough areas at the knees and ankles are also found to create an erogenous sensation if stimulated with soft caresses.

2

SENSUAL MASSAGE IN SEX THERAPY

Sensual Massage plays an important role in Sex Therapy these days. This has manifold effects on the sexual well-being of the person, but it is mainly used to stimulate and enhance their libido (positive response to sexual stimuli. It is also done by professionals on men who have premature ejaculation issues.

The use of Sensual Genital Massage refers to physicians' use to treat women having Female Hysteria. This was popular as a treatment until finally, the patients were referred to midwives. However, it was time-consuming, and the patients needed treatment regularly.

Some techniques have been derived from research that enhances orgasm in both men and women. One such technique is called Extended Orgasm. It does not come under normal orgasms but can be explained as more intense sensations that last anywhere from some minutes to an hour or more. In addition, the orgasms have been.

Neo Tantra

This is the Western modification of Tantric Sex. Tantric Sex is all about elevating sexual satisfaction to a spiritual level, whereas the former is not that much into spiritual attainment. After thorough research on the Buddhist and Hindu Tantra, the Western Neo-Tantra has come to be.

It involves all the rituals of the traditional one and has brought forth many unorthodox movements. There is also a famous school of thought called Sex Magic.

3

HOW IS SENSUAL MASSAGE DONE?

Sensual Massage can be done alone or with a partner. It can be used for various reasons, the main ones being:

1. Reaching or enhancing orgasms
2. A heightened level of foreplay

Controlled Orgasms

Controlled orgasms heighten the level of sexual release to a heightened level and even may never stimulate levels of consciousness. This can be done alone or with the help of a partner. It is a technique of maintaining the highest level of arousal for extended periods. Although the climax plateau of men is lower than that of women, using this technique, men can go for repeated coitus without the delay of refractory periods that come after normal orgasms. It is a series of peaked sexual stimuli without a complete release of sexual tension. When the final release is made, the orgasm attained is so high that it results in multiple orgasms and states of mind that can be called Euphoric.

ORGASM CONTROL WITH A PARTNER

This is a sex game that involves sensual massage as the foreplay, building up the tension, and giving full control of the orgasm to the partner. The receiver is made to reach the level of stimulation just below that orgasm's Point of No Return. This is done by altering the speed and stimulation of the sexual activity involved. This is done multiple times by giving small gaps that bring the heightened tension level to almost zero. All the tensions that have been 'denied' build up and the final orgasm(s) will be of a much-heightened level.

MASTURBATION:

This is practiced to attain higher levels of orgasmic release or to prolong the coitus with a partner. People usually follow a masturbation 'exercise' as they fully control regulating their peaks and troughs of sexual tension. There are two ways of attaining this.

1. Edging: This is done by letting go of all stimulation just before sexual release letting the stimulated tension go all the way to zero, and building it up again.
2. Surfing: In this variation, there is no complete letting go but continue with the stimulation at a reduced level of intensity.

4

BEGINNERS GUIDE TO SENSUAL MASSAGE

Now that you know the benefits and techniques involved in Sensual Massage let's look at how to give it to your partner:

Toolkit:

1. A Massage Bed: Since it will involve a lot of sexual stimulation and gaps that reduce tension, it is best to give the massage to your partner on a bed. A bed at the proper height will also be easy on your back as you will not have to strain your pose or muscles.
2. A Pillow: Your partner has to shift from a supine position to a flat on back position. When your partner takes a supine position, a pillow under the knees is very relaxing, and when lying flat on the tummy, a pillow under the head is to be offered.
3. Thick Blanket: If you offer massage in a setting like a fireplace or don't have a massage bed, a blanket will come in handy.
4. Scented candles and incense sticks also create an

ambiance that gets cozy with soft music playing in the background.
5. Last but not least, a selection of lubricants. Though you can give a sensual massage with a base oil, it is much better to give one using an Aromatherapy oil. Some also have an aphrodisiac effect but pay close attention to the dilution of the Aromatherapy Oils as some may be harmful and cause allergic reactions.

THE BASICS:

1. Arrange a room that is cozily warm. A massage is just not it f the person feels cold. Slow music, reduced lighting, and some fragrances will set the complete mood for you.
2. Let them feel that you are offering something special as a token of love.
3. Always start with the person lying flat on the back with their head resting on a pillow of a folded blanket. This is done so that there is no direct stimulation to the genitals at the start and also to build up the mood. People are less shy to start with a back massage than a frontal one.
4. Apply a little bit of warm oil in your hands and start massaging their back. Slow unbroken kneads or circles will do the job of warming up their mood.
5. The order of a massage is:
6. Back
7. Legs
8. Turnover and massage the feet
9. Legs
10. Arms
11. Shoulder
12. Scalp

13. Breasts and pubic region
14. You should not have a fixed schedule as 2 minutes to each part if your partner wants a certain area to be massaged more than be in the giving mood. They eventually will be in the mood for a much more intense massage.

NURU MASSAGE:

This Japanese form of massage tops the list as it is done body to body. It creates more closeness among partners as the massage is not done with the hands but with the whole body and creates a lot of intimacy and heightened levels of sexual stimulation.

Nuru means 'Slippery' and contrary to the general rule in massage 'not to overdo the lubricant', this uses a generous amount on the body, and there are also special gels in the market.

This massage is done in the nude i.e., both the partners are nude, and the closest you can get to penetration intimacy is present.

Start by applying the gel on your body, allowing a teasing glance to your partner and stimulating yourself. Pour a generous gel helping and apply it on your partner with your hands first. Then massage their muscles with your forearms. Next, go side by side, continue with the sliding motion, and mount on your partner. You can use your buttocks and groin area to massage them before going completely body to body. The best part of a Nuru Massage is taking turns in the same session.

5

GELS AND OILS USED FOR SENSUAL MASSAGE

Though there are a lot of Aromatherapy Oils in the market, they are not solely for sensual Massages, so here are some other gels and oils that you can use.

1. Honey: Honey has a lot of health benefits and about 190 nutrients that are nourishing for the body as well as detoxifying. It can be directly applied to wounds and gashes. It is also considered an aphrodisiac, and you can use your mouth or tongue to massage those special places of your partner.
2. Lavender: This soothes the muscles and completely relaxes your partner. Inhaling the fumes of this oil also relaxes the mind and opens up your partner's mood for a sexual massage.
3. Aloe Vera: If you want to infuse a lot of health benefits in your Sensual Massage, then Aloe Vera would come in the top list. It contains over 200 nutritive ingredients and is antibiotic and antifungal, to name a few benefits.
4. Orange Oil: This helps in the circulation of blood in

the body and is especially stimulating if applied at Erogenous Zones of the body.

5. Peppermint: Mint and menthol have been long related to sexual activity. The smallest suggestion of it will heighten the mood. It also relaxes the muscles.

6. Rosemary: Rosemary is a muscle relaxant and best to use if your partner is tired or just not at his best.

7. Melilot: Melilot is also an effective relaxant and can relax your partner's mood.

6

SENSUAL MASSAGE TECHNIQUES

FOR MEN:

1. Begin with the head. All men love when their head is fondled. Start at the scalp and go down the head in soft circular motions.
2. Use a blend of oil known for its relaxing aroma, like Sandalwood.
3. Take a liberal helping of oil. It is best to patch test the oil if you have an Essential Oil kit, as some may cause allergic reactions.
4. Move slowly down from the head to the neck and then to the shoulder and to the back.
5. Listen to feedback from him. If he wants a bit more attention at a specific spot, linger there a bit longer. Men usually love long caresses to the head.
6. Massage downwards as this is good for improving blood circulation. Use the type of pressure he likes (evident in his feedback). There are no hard and fast rules in Sensual Massage.
7. There are chances that he falls asleep that is normal

and if you wish to wake him do so after 20-25 minutes. He will have had a very refreshing sleep and will feel rejuvenated.

Trigger Zones in Men:

Paying special attention to 'Trigger Zones' will heighten the efficiency of a sensual massage.

1. The Lips. The lower lip and the curve that leads down to the chin is a very sensitive zone. Kissing his lip and using your tongue to caress it will make him come to his mood fast. This is especially good if he has fallen asleep and you need to wake him up after the 20 minutes gap.
2. The Neck: Use a feather or a soft kiss to stimulate nerve endings behind his neck (nape). Continue the motion unbroken along his collar bone and under Adam's apple.
3. The Nipples: A man's nipples are just as sensitive as a woman's, and newer studies show that they are more sensitive than a woman's. Licking on the areola and rolling his nipples with your tongue is stimulating.
4. The Inner Thighs. These are very sensitive to touch as they join at the pubic area. Slow circular motions at the inner thigh and a spreading motion that goes upward and back again with a random caress at the perineum are a sure tease for any man.

FOR WOMEN:

1. Start with moderate pressure on the lower back, avoid

the spine, and work up in a gentle elliptical round spanning her back.
2. Use your thumbs at the shoulders, massaging away any knots if you notice them. Always use slow pressure on the shoulders.
3. Go down her arm and massage her palms, rolling each finger slowly between your palms.
4. Women love foot massages, and paying special attention can make you a winner if she finds it tickly to go slower with a bit more pressure.
5. Listen for feedback moans or non-verbal signs like her body rising for contact with yours.
6. Gliding movements on her sides with a slow teasing touch at the sides of her breast are very stimulating as these are soft and sensitive areas.
7. When massaging her lying flat on her tummy, make slow inward motions at her inner thighs up to just under her pubic area and then down.
8. Make her roll over and massage her feet and legs. She will feel relaxed and open for many intimate touches.

7

ADVANCED SENSUAL MASSAGE

Once you have done some basic massages to your partner and it has become a regular thing in your love life, then it's time to go in advanced mode. Discuss it with your partner before going into this mode.

YONI MASSAGE

1. Yoni Massage: Yoni is the Sanskrit term for Vagina. This adds a spiritual twist to the massage and is about respecting her sacredness through reverence to her genitalia.

The woman lies on her back with pillows at her head and buttocks. Her legs are spread comfortably, and her Yoni is in full view. Her partner sits directly in front and between her legs. Inhale through your nose and exhale from your mouth. The body is let to shed out negativity as each part is relaxed. Starting at the head and going all the way down to the legs. Each breath relaxes each part of the body.

Apply a bit of oil to your palms and softly massage the inner thighs with alternating long and short and varied pressure up and down her inner thighs. Softly caress the Yoni in an up and down motion at first and then spread the lips a bit. Pay attention to the outer folds of her Yoni and once in her Yoni, look for feedback signs of what sensations she loves best. Apply a bit more oil before proceeding to her clitoris. Alternate touches and pressure and try softly pressing it with your fingers.

Yoni Massage is not focused on orgasm but an intimate bond between you and her. Prolong the session as long as she wants it to. Get to know her limit of arousal. If she reaches an orgasm, hug her as close and warm as possible and enjoy the feeling of your heart reflecting on the massage. You must maintain eye contact throughout the massage.

PROSTATE MASSAGE

1. Prostate Massage: This is commonly done on men. The prostate is the area surrounding his bladder and urethra. It is usually stimulated through the anus as it can be found near the anterior part of the rectum.

The person needs to empty his bowels, wash the anus with warm water and soap, and clean it a bit deeper than usual. This is done with fingers and surgical gloves, and a lot of lubricants are advised. Never use your fingers directly as they can tear the soft tissues in the rectum.

. . .

Have him lie flat on a bed with his buttocks in a clean view. After he takes some deep breath and feels relaxed, inserts your finger slowly and deep until you reach a knot in the tunnel.

Use slow circular motions. Slowly increase the pressure and decrease it if he feels any discomfort. Some men become intensely aroused, but a prostate massage is done best if kept to 15 minutes or until he asks to stop.

Never make Prostate Massage a routine, leading to serious medical conditions. Once in two weeks is the best to engage in it.

The End.

Did you like this book? Then you'll LOVE Perfect Essential Oils: What You Wish You Knew About Essential Oils

Click here to start reading Perfect Essential Oils NOW!

https://books2read.com/u/mBwALR

SNEAK PEEK - CHAPTER 1

Did you like this book? Then you'll LOVE Perfect Essential Oils: What You Wish You Knew About Essential Oils

Click here to start reading Perfect Essential Oils NOW!

https://books2read.com/u/mBwALR

Essential Oils.

A massage is a common form of treating the body, therapeutically or otherwise, using a body part to enhance or relax other body parts. You see this in all cultures and regions of the world.

The word means to 'knead' whether it be the French word massage, the Arabic 'massa', or even the Greek 'masso'.

People have often wondered how a relaxing and comforting treatment cures ailments of the body and mind. Ancient Ayurvedic texts explain toxins accumulate daily in the issues, and a massage dissolves them and slowly removes them from the system.

Ayurveda also goes on and recommends 'Abhyanga' or oil massage as part of everyday life. The texts go on and list out the benefits. Some of them are:

It is nourishing to the body
Reduces fatigue
Stimulates relaxed and deep sleep
Provides stamina
Improves the complexion and luster of the skin
Detoxifies
Improves longevity
Increased circulation to the nerve endings
Toning of the whole muscle structure
Soothes the nerves
Lubricates joints
Improves mental alertness

These are some of the benefits that are seen among people who indulge in a massage daily.

Massages serve many purposes, from treating an ailing part of the body to enhancing the reflexes to a warm relaxing, or sensual one. It is usually done by using both hands, but nowadays, sensual massages involve body o body massage.

When a massage is applied, there are many things to consider: the ambiance, the pressure used, the body condition, and even the medium used. We will be mainly discussing the medium here in this book as it is of utmost importance.

Most massages are done using base oils. These are good as they nourish the skin and act as medicine for most skin ailments. The most popular ones are Jojoba, Wheat Germ, and Olive oil. These are added to any primary oil to improve its medicinal value.

Essential oils differ from Base oils as the former are derived from extracting concentrated essences from seeds, fruit, or other plant sources. As a result, these double in their therapeutic value also.

End of Sneak Peek.

Did you like this book? Then you'll LOVE Perfect Essential Oils: What You Wish You Knew About Essential Oils

Click here to start reading Perfect Essential Oils NOW!

https://books2read.com/u/mBwALR

www.ingramcontent.com/pod-product-compliance
Lightning Source LLC
LaVergne TN
LVHW021748060526
838200LV00052B/3531